It Is All Abou

How to Eat What You Want and Lose Weight Immediately

By Gabrielle Hollis

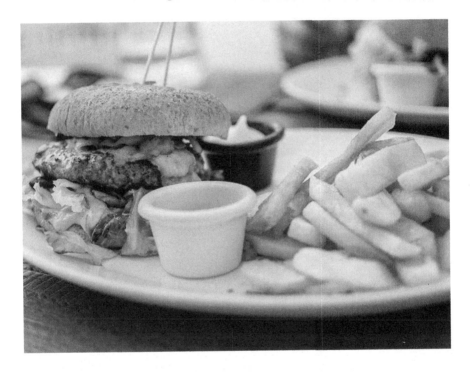

Table of Contents

Introduction

Have you been thinking about losing weight lately? Is your weight becoming a huge problem to your health and self-esteem? Do you want to lose that weight safely? Well, worry no more! Losing weight is one of the greatest thing that many people often consider to be daunting! But the truth is losing weight is part of weight management. You may be thinking, but how can that be? Well, having too much weight often is not good for your health. It simply increases your chance of developing such diseases as heart problems, type 2 diabetes, certain types of cancer as well as high blood pressure among others.

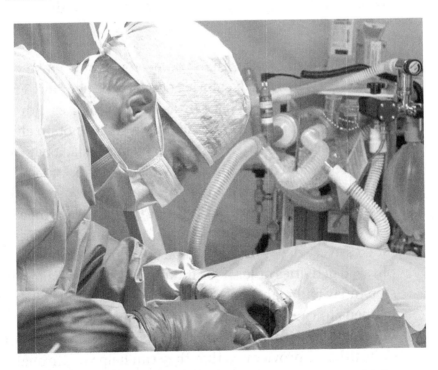

In other cases, research has shown that being overweight can be a predisposing factor to certain conditions such as osteoarthritis, respiratory diseases as well as sleep apnea among others. Being overweight is something that can make you feel sad or be treated by others in a way that is demeaning. You do not want that, right?

There are so many ways in which you can shed off that weight and take back your self-esteem. I want you to understand that you are in control of every decision that you make. You can lose weight by simply making smart choices about your lifestyle. What you eat and what you do with your body! Choosing to eat fewer calories and exercising regularly are one of the most common ways in which you can lose weight. So many people say that they have no control of what they eat. Others say that when they feel sad, they find it calming to indulge in high calorie food and snacks. Trust me, just like you reach out to that bowl of ice cream of chocolate, you can choose not to by replacing it with a healthy alternative.

Eating so much calories than you need will only make you overweight. How much calories do you take per day? Try as much as you can to cut back by about 500 calories. For instance, if you have been indulging in sodas, potato chips and chocolate bars, try to cut down by one soda, a bag of potato chips and a chocolate bar which are 150, 150 and 250 calories respectively. For many people, this may seem like a slow way to lose weight, but it is not the only way you can lose weight. While you are cutting down on these calorie intakes every day, you also will be engaging your body in physical activities at least 30 minutes every day. Take a bold step today and make lifelong lifestyle choices and watch what happens to your weight. Ensure that you share the information we present here with your dietician, nutritionist or healthcare provider so that they can help you through your weight loss journey in achieving every goal in the right way possible for you.

If you speak to a health professional, they will tell that losing weight gradually is the way to go. The main reason for losing weight gradually but within the shortest time is the fact that it is highly likely that that weight will stay off. If you indulge in things that will make you lose weight fast, trust me, you will lose muscles, water and bones rather than shed off extra fat that you do not need.

According to the Academy of Nutrition and Dietetics, it is healthy for anyone trying to lose weight to aim for at least 1-2 pounds per week. Stay away from anything that may seem too good to be true. It is best if you can base your weight loss on milestones you can stick to for a very long period of time. You would like you weight loss regime to be part of your lifestyle, right? That is the way to go! So, what are you waiting for? Come with me and let's shed excess weight, shall we?

So, what is the plan?

Well, ever heard of the saying 'garbage in, garbage out?' This is also applicable when it comes to weight loss. This simply means, calories in, calories out! In other words, you need to burn as much calories as you eat and drink. However, it is not that simple.

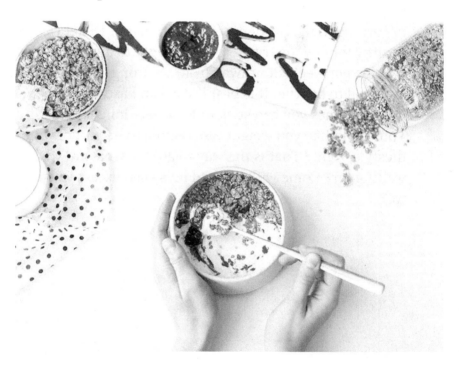

What really matters is your metabolism (the manner in which your body burns calories into fuel). This means that, if you cut too much calories than the body requires, it can have adverse effects on you. You can end up slowing down your metabolism and that can be a bad thing as it may cause you to fall short on important nutrients.

Just to highlight this, there are several ways in which you can achieve this. Some of these ways include; cutting back on small portions, figuring out how many calories you get in a usual day and then trimming back on them a little, reading food labels just to know how many calories there are per serving and so you can make informed decisions as well as drinking a lot of water, which can be filling and reduces your urge for food.

Another tip that I will start with before we delve deeper into important factors we need to discuss about weight loss is ensuring that you get accountability and support. There are so many applications that you can use to keep track of your eating and how many calories you consume and how many you lose every day. So many people today have smartphones and if you have one, then you can download one of the many apps in the market to help you keep up with the plan. You could also use a pen-and-paper food journal so that you keep in record everything that you eat and when you eat them.

One of the best ways in which you can stay motivated is having people around you who can cheer you on and stay by your side to make sure that you are following through with your plan and that you are working towards achieving your weight loss goals. So, instead of struggling on your own, ask your family and friends to support you in your journey to losing weight. The other thing you can do is joining a weight loss group. Here, you can meet other people who are trying to lose weight as you do. There are so many reasons why people decide to lose weight, and you could learn a lot their journey as well. Trust me, their encouragements can be very contagious-but in a very good way!

Chapter 1

Finding Your Drive

Do you know what drives you to eat? Well, at the very least, one of the most important things that you have to understand is that food is fuel. It is the thing that gives you energy to do a number of tasks and activities each day. Your body and brain need that energy. Unfortunately, there are so few people that eat because s reason. I was one of them until I made a decision to lose weight and adopt a healthy lifestyle like you are trying to do as well. You will find plenty of food at social gatherings at home and even at work during meetings, birthday parties among other events. This is where so many of us turn to just when we have had a very rough day.

It is important that you know what it is that drives you into eating. Especially when you are not hungry! Having knowledge of the things that make us eat when we are not hungry plays a critical role when it comes to weight loss because then, we can have a plan for these moments.

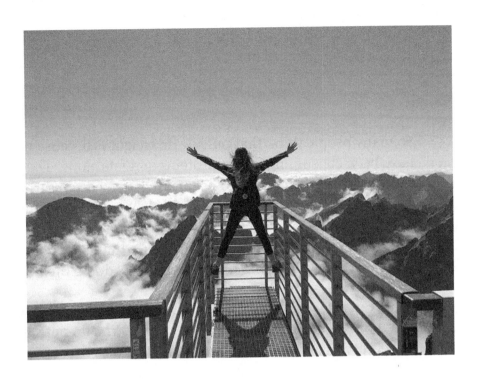

The very first step is determining what is your trigger. Is it anger, stress, depression, anxiety or something else happening in your life? Or is it that you turn to food as a reward for something good that you have achieved?

Once you have this, the next thing is for you to take note of it when it happens. When these feelings come up, do you have a plan? Is there something that you can do rather than eating? Could you maybe call a friend, take a walk or even do some chores in the house so that you are distracted? Whatever it is, try as much as you can to stick to the plan and then once you have achieved it, you can reward yourself with many different choices other than food. You can buy that dress you have been admiring in the clothing store, or you can treat yourself to a spa among others.

Now try to reset what you eat and when you eat it

So many people think that putting on weight is because you have been consuming lots of proteins and fats alone. They think it is because of eating beef and meaty foods. Yes, these foods may contribute to significant weight gain, but going vegan or gluten-free will not be your only solution. Interesting enough, there is a high chance that you might end up keeping the extra pounds rather than shedding them off.

However, what really makes sense is being able to cut down or cut out these excess calories completely. You do not want any empty calories! So, how do you do this?

Limit added sugars

Added sugars are those that you find in cakes, cookies, sugar-sweetened drinks among other foods and snacks. These often are loaded with unnecessary and very unhealthy sugars. They are not the sugars that you would naturally find in fruits or other plant-based products. The truth is, these sugary foods have lots of calories loaded in them. Therefore, if you are going to make weight loss the number one priority, then you have to make a bold decision to spend less than 10% of your daily calorie-intake on added sugars.

Be very choosy about carbs

This means that you have to make a decision what carbs you will consume and which ones you will not. You also have to decide how much you will take. The best moves you can make is taking those carbs that are very low on the glycemic index. For instance, instead of taking potatoes, you can choose to replace them with asparagus which has a very low glycemic index.

Another important tip is that you can eat whole grains which are a better choice than processed foods. Remember that, when foods are processed, so many essential nutrients are removed. Such nutrients include but are not limited to iron, fiber as well as B vitamins. These nutrients may be added back especially in enriched breads.

Include proteins

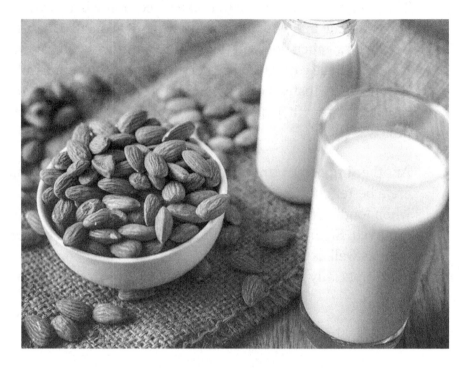

Proteins are a very healthy part of a balanced diet. It is proteins that play a central role in ensuring that you keep your muscles in check while keeping you satisfied. If you are a vegan or a vegetarian, there are so many sources that you can choose from including; nuts, soy and beans. On the other hand, if you are not either of these, then you should be able to consume lean meat, fish, poultry and dairy products.

The most surprising thing that research has revealed is that many Americans prefer getting their proteins from lean meat. However, it is important that you insist on consuming white meat in place of red meats for health reasons. Another important thing to bear in mind is that your protein needs often is dependent on such factors as age, gender as well as how active you are.

Insist on good fats

It does not mean that all fats are bad. There are very good fats that your body and brain need. Therefore, it is important that you make good friends with good fats so that they can help you stay full and less like you are dieting.

Some of the best choices that you can integrate into your plan include; seeds, nuts, coconut as well as olive oils among others. These are the fat sources that are loaded with unsaturated fats which includes poly-and mono-unsaturated fats.

Fill up on fiber

You can fill up with fiber from vegetables, fruits as well as whole grains. Just know that you can fill up a lot of fiber from plant foods. Different plant foods have different amounts of fiber. There are those that have more fiber than others and you can comfortably incorporate thins into your diet. Some of the fiber sources that have a lot in them include green peas, lime beans, artichokes, lentils and broccoli. In the fruits family, you can get lots of fiber from raspberries which is at the very top of the list.

Eat small portions every often

You may be wondering 'how do you expect me to lose weight if I am going to be eating often?' Well, am not saying that you consume so much calories at the same go. If you are going to keep your tummy full and keep anger at bay, you need to eat small portions 5-6 times a day. This is very important especially when it comes to losing weight.

You can achieve this by simply spreading the calories equally across all these mini-meals. You could also make some meals bigger than others but at the end of the day, you will have taken the *required number of calories and nothing more than it*. Plan portions so that you do not end up consuming more than your bargain.

Meal replacements

Did you know that you can replace some meals with more healthy options? This is how you can be able to keep your calorie-intake in check. Making meal replacements play a very critical role in weight loss as they are very convenient and they get rid of the need for people to guess how much each meal has in terms of calories, hence making dieting effortless. The most important thing that you have to bear in mind is that you have to change your eating habits so that you keep that weight off in case you go off the meal replacements.

Watch closely what you drink

According to research, one of the easiest ways in one can lose weight is by cutting down on liquid calories. These are sodas, alcohol, juices among others. The truth is, it is very easy to fall in the habit of consuming sugar-sweetened drinks. Rather than doing this, you can simply replace them with sugar-free or zero-calorie drinks that include black coffee, lemon water or even unsweetened tea.

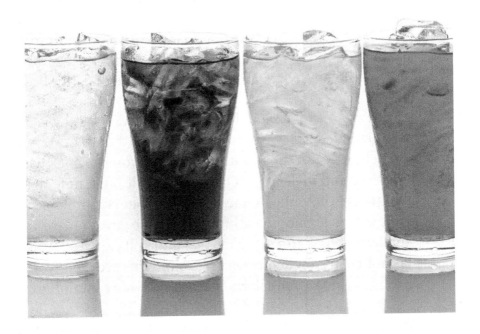

Note that, when you take diet drinks, they save you a hell lots of calories compared to taking sugary beverages. Do not make your plan backfire just because you think that you can replace the drinks with a cookie just because you feel hungry.

So, should you fast?

Well, this is one of the most frequently asked questions that people are interested in knowing the answer. Well, I have a friend that was trying to lose weight and they thought that they could do this by fasting so that they could just drop off as much pounds as they possibly could within the shortest time possible. Well, if you are thinking the same, think again!

According to experts and health nutritionists, fasting is not recommended as a weight loss regime. Rather than starving yourself, why not try an eating plan that you can stick with over time and make it part of your lifestyle. Just note that not all fasts are the same. Some fasts are about skipping meals while others are about eating every single day. You are wondering, how can someone fast and still eat. Well, there has not been so much research around this area, but you can fast by keeping your calorie intake to the bear minimum.

You will realize that, during the early days of your fast, you will get angry and even grumpy. In other, you may feel like you are constipated. During this time, you may feel like you do not have the energy to get work done, physically. Ensure that you take plenty of water and have a multivitamin supplement. You also need to run this by your doctor to ensure that you can do this. Otherwise, if you are on medication, you may need to make sure that you go through proper examination and advice by a health professional. Just remember that, even though you are on a fast, you have to adjust your eating habits once the fast is over.

Regardless of how you kick-start your weight loss, one thing that you have to remember is that if you want to keep that weight off, you have to adopt long-lasting lifestyle adjustments. This can be in the form of a healthy eating plan and a physical activity. If you are not so sure about where to start, don't worry we will be discussing this in the next chapters.

Chapter 2

Reasons and Benefits of Weight Loss

Trust me, carrying around so much weight can be very uncomfortable-hell, even depressing. Based on a report by the Centers for Disease Control (CDC) the rates at which obesity is skyrocketing in the US is quite alarming. This is because, as of 2010, more than 1/3 of American adults were considered to be obese based on their Basal Metabolic Index (BMI) which was greater than 30.

BMI=Weight (pounds)/Height (inches squared)

To calculate your body mass, start by multiplying your weight in pounds by 703. Then calculate your height in inches squared. After which, divide the number you get from your weight by the one you get from your height.

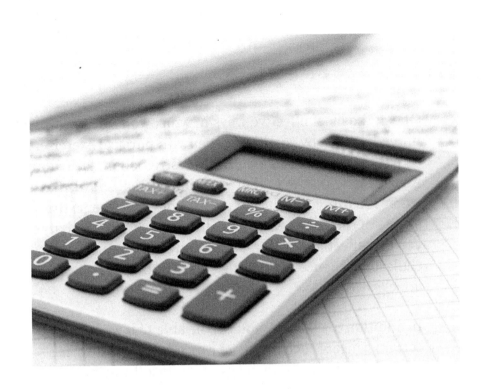

If your BMI>= 30 you are obese

BMI>=25-29 you are overweight

BMI>=18.5-24 you are normal

BMI<= 18 you are underweight.

One thing that you have to understand is that obesity is a very serious condition and can lead to a series of very serious health issues. Therefore, it will really help if you pay attention to the information that we have already discussed in the above chapter.

Benefits of weight loss

One of the most effective ways in which you can lose weight immediately is by combining diet with physical exercise, rather than depending on calorie restriction in itself alone. According to research, there is evidence that shows that when you exercise, you can prevent or even reverse the effects of certain diseases. It is through physical activity that you can effectively lower your blood pressure and levels of cholesterol, hence preventing such conditions as heart attacks.

In addition to exercise, you can be able to lower your risk for certain cancers such as breast cancer and colon cancer among others. It simply plays a significant role in contributing towards helping you get back your sense of self-confidence and self-esteem, hence lowering the rates of anxiety and depression.

You need to engage in physical activity so that you can lose weight and maintain weight loss. It is through physical activity that you can increase metabolism and the number of calories you burn every day. It also is very important in helping you maintain and increase a lean body mass, which helps boost the number of calories you burn/day.

So, how much exercise if required to lose weight?

In order to reap the benefits of exercise, it is very important that you perform some form of aerobic exercise. Least 3-4 times every week. Each aerobic exercise should last about 20-30 minutes per session if you really want to shed off those extra pounds. You can also incorporate 15 minutes if exercise such as cycling and walking every day so that you can burn an extra 100 or more calories. If you burn a minimum of 700 calories a week, this equals about 10 lbs. of weight loss annually.

Imagine if you worked extra hard to increase your weight loss beyond this bear minimum, what weight would that be? How would you feel about yourself? You can do it. Just take a bold step and make decision. Remember, everything is under your control as far as weight loss is concerned.

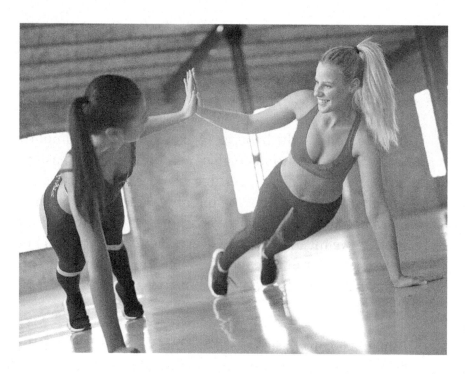

How do you calculate your target heart rate?

In order to enjoy all the health benefits that exercise has to offer, you have to ensure that you blend in some high intensity exercises. For you to have an idea of how hard re working, you have to keep checking your heart rate. To do this, you can use the formula;

Target heart rate= 60 to 80 % of (220-Age)

Ensure that you consult with your trainer or a healthcare team provider so that they can help you determine the best intensity workout you can engage in every day. If you have special health concerns such as a heart condition, injury, have been on a surgery recent, diabetes or any other condition, you have to ensure that you speak to your physician before you can enroll on health fitness program.

Think about it!

When you make the decision to make exercise a part of your lifestyle, trust me, you will shed that weight and take control of your body and weight again. The total amount of exercises that you choose to engage in every day matters a lot. This is the reason why every single milestone you make, however small it is in your daily routine will make a great difference in your waistline.

Take time to walk around, take a ride on your bike around the block or your neighborhood as well as when you are running errands. Rather than taking the elevator to your office or to your appointment, choose to take the stairs. Instead of parking at your destination, you can choose to park further so that you can take the remaining time to walk that distance. Whatever it is, you always have the choice, and you can choose to make take sedentary lifestyles off the list by making some bold health moves.

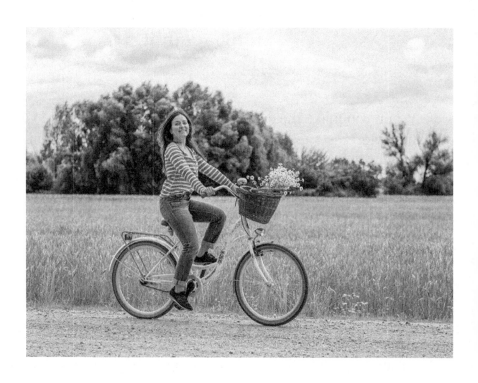

Before you get started on that exercise program, ensure that you talk to your doctor especially in cases where you would like to engage in vigorous exercise. I cannot emphasize this enough. If have certain high-risk conditions such as a heart, lung, kidney disease, diabetes or arthritis, making healthy moves by enrolling in an exercise program is good, but not without a greenlight from your health advisor.

If you also have been inactive for a very long period of time or have recently quit smoking or you just found out that you are overweight, ensure that you speak to a doctor before you can engage in physical exercise that is quite vigorous. This is because, when starting a new program that the body is not used to, it is important that you understand the various signals that your body will give. That way, you will know when something is wrong or when you have to keep pushing yourself until you get an improvement. However, if you push yourself too hard, this can lead to injury. If you experience any pain or shortness of breath, you should stop exercising immediately.

Why should you lose weight?

Weight management is one of the rising concerns in the health care industry with doctors, weight loss providers and nutritionists encouraging people to lead a life characterized by an adequate intake of balanced diet coupled with physical activity. Having weight loss as one of your plans to lead a healthy life is very important for so many reasons.

These reasons include;

Less pressure on the joints

One of the most common problems that people who are obese is experiencing joint pains around their knee region. This is quite obvious; too much weight puts so much pressure on the joints resulting into sever pain. Apart from the pain around the knees, back, elbows and ankles, weight also results in pain due to weight stress. If you follow a weight management guide, you will not only be able to shed off lots of pounds from the body, but also build muscle that is able to bear the weight of the body much comfortably.

Sleep apnea

This may sound weird to you, but it is absolutely true. Having too much weight can lead to development of a sleep disorder commonly referred to as sleep apnea. In other words, you do not get enough good quality sleep as a result of blocked airways during sleep. During sleep, an obese person may not be able to sleep well because they cannot breathe well and so they keep waking up many times. Because of inadequate sleep, you could also develop a disturbance of the metabolism hence resulting into slow rate that eventually causes fat accumulation. Indeed, it is important to note that sleep is very important for your health and this is exactly how!

Strengthen the immune system

Having the right body weight is very important for your immune system. You may be wondering 'but how is this linked to the immune system?' Well, when we pay a close attention to our lifestyle to ensure that we are healthy by taking fruits, vegetables, water and other important nutrients, we are providing the body with all the nutrients it needs to build a strong immune system. This means that, you develop a strong body that is able to fight off infections and stay healthy.

Fertility

According to research, it is clear that over 1/3 or adults in the US are obese as we already mentioned in chapter above. This could explain the reason why so many adult women within the child bearing age are having a difficulty conceiving and getting children. The truth is, obese people have a difficulty conceiving and when they do, the experience a lot of complications during childbirth that either puts the child in danger or their lives in danger.

As a matter of fact, obesity is the major factor contributing to poly-Cystic Syndrome, a condition that affects fertility in women. On the other hand, obese women have a difficulty having natural child birth. And because of this, they end up using C-section as the only solution to childbirth.

Appearance and self-esteem

Along with the major health concerns that obesity possess on a person, the truth is obesity is one of the reasons why people want to look good. Obesity often brings down someone's self-esteem and rips them of their self-confidence both at home and at work.

There are so many places, though not mentioned out a loud that cannot offer you a job just because you are obese. Though this may sound like discrimination, the truth is, being allowed to work in such places will not only strip you of your self-confidence, but also make you look bad. We all want to look beautiful like those models we watch on TV, and the only way to get started in adopting a weight loss management plan that works for you. The secret is for you to start now and watch what weight loss does to your self-confidence, esteem and personality in general-fire!

So, what really is the role of medical weight management?

Well, let me start here by stating that the idea of losing weight is fantastic and positive. It is liberating to note that one is concerned about how they look as well as the health and well-being of their body. Losing weight is about eating in moderation and indulging in physical exercise so that we can build our muscle and take good care of our tissues.

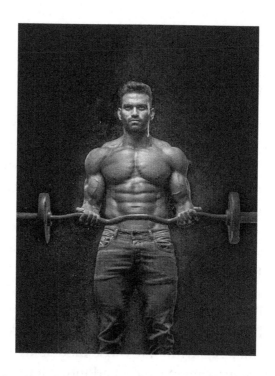

With the help of a weight loss clinic, you can be able to achieve the best results by adopting an effective strategy on weight management. You will be able to get guidelines on; customized diet plan and body assessments, medical weight loss works up, development of healthy eating habits, expert structured fitness program as well as regaining control over your health and confidence.

Chapter 3

Cardio-Exercises for Weight Loss

Regardless of what exercise you choose, the most important thing that you have to bear in mind with is that if it has to work, you have to do it. this is the very reason why experts recommend that you pick exercises that you can enjoy doing. This is very important in ensuring that you stick to a regular routine.

Irrespective of what exercise program you choose to implement, you have to ensure that aerobics is part of them. Aerobics are simply cardiovascular exercises. They play a significant role in getting your heart rate up as well as increasing the rate at which blood is pumped.

They often include jogging, walking, cycling, dancing and swimming. You could also do your workouts on a treadmill, stair stepped as well as elliptical among others. Let's have a look at some that you can incorporate in your exercise routine.

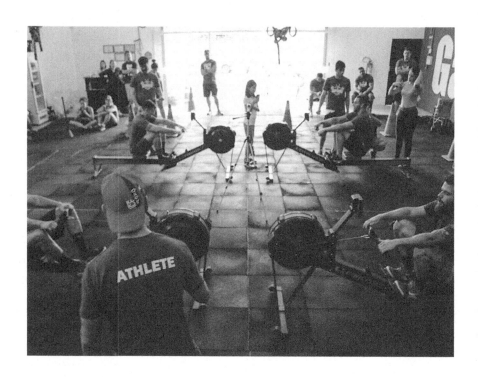

Sprinting

This is one of the top most cardio exercises that serve as an excellent way to burn calories in the least amount of time possible. Whether you are sprinting on a treadmill, outside or wherever you feel much comfortable, you are sure to shed off that extra weight fast. The good thing with sprints is the fact that you do not need any equipment because you can do them anywhere.

Sprinting is quite simple, and you get to burn as much calories as you can. To lose that weight fast, this should be at the top of your list. While you still lose weight while running and jogging, increasing the speed and intensity at which you do this really pays off. The best part of this exercise is the fact that it leaves no muscles unscathed. If you are looking to gain back your six pack, then go full steam on this and watch what happens.

If you are sprinting outside on a running track, try sprinting one lap and jogging another lap. Keep alternating this for as long as you can and you will lose as much weight as you can. On the other hand, if you are sprinting on a treadmill, it is important that you do an all-out-sprint for about half an hour, then slowing down and jogging for like a minute before repeating. If you have access to a stadium, you can try running up the stairs as fast as you can, then jog or walk on your way down. While at it ensure that you really lift those knees as high as you can so that your glutes get some great action and hence, build sprinter power within no time.

High intensity interval training

This is also referred to as HIIT. His exercise gives you a well-rounded workout while ensuring that you burn those fats and calories and shed off lots of weight. This exercise can vary from 500 an hour to over 1500 + calories an hour for an average weight person. They are really great considering the intensity of each exercise. When you pair body weight movements with weighted movements as well as traditional cardio factors, you are sure to achieve the perfect fat burner.

Rowing

Do you know of any collegiate rower? Well, if you are then I bet you are seriously envious of those athletic V-cut frame as I am. If you are going to shed off that extra weight, it is better if you have rowing at the top of the list. This is because it offers you a great way to integrate the upper and the lower parts of the body in a moderately less stressful manner especially on the joints and the ligaments. It also is a great way to really work your posterior chain. On a rowing machine, you can burn an average of 800 calories/hour. However, if you increase the intensity and couple it with short sprints, trust me, you will burn over 1000 calories/hour as fast as you can.

While rowing, it is important that you keep your chest up and use the rest of your body. Do not let your arms do all the work. Try as much as you can to use your legs to achieve motion and keep it going.

Swimming

People think that someone who is overweight or obese cannot swim but they will sink. Well, truth be told, swimming is more like a mind exercise. If you are going to fit in that designer model bikini, swimming is one of the exercises that will help you shed as much weight as you can. It is a total-body workout that begin as soon as you start treading water. When swimming, you are constantly fighting the forces of gravity. This means that, your muscles are working as hard as they can to keep you afloat. According to research, *swimming just for a minute burns 14 calories*. Incredible, right? Get swimming and shed off that weight.

The other trick when swimming is the types of strokes that you employ. For instance, if you are using the breast stroke, you will burn less calories compared to using the butterfly strokes. Therefore, be sure to incorporate the different types of strokes to achieve maximum weight loss within the shortest time possible.

One thing I would like you to remember when swimming is that if you are going to lose weight, you need to tread water so that you can burn lots of calories. You can achieve this by simply doing a couple of laps and having a water-treading interval in between. If you can swim at a high level, then swim as fast as you can for as long as you can. If you are not much of a swimmer, then you can do swim intervals where you swim fast down the length of the pool and back and have slower swim intervals in between throughout the entire duration of the workout.

Cycling

In most of the gyms, stationery bikes are a mainstay. However, there is a reason why not many people are on the queue waiting for them. The truth is, if it is going to help you shed off that weight, you have to be willing to really take it on a spin. In other words, you have to really go at a high rate of intensity. You cannot burn calories when you are cycling slowly while surfing your smartphone! For a vigorous indoor cycling exercise, you can burn at least **1,150 calories an hour** while a moderate ride will burn about half of that amount.

When you incorporate interval stationery cycling, you maximize your chances of burning as much calories as you can within minimum time. The trick is for you to keep the intensity high enough for a couple of minutes before slowing down and continually repeating this for as long as you can.

Kettlebells

While this exercise is not a cardio-only workout, the impact it has as far as burning calories goes is too high to keep it off this list. It simply combines the best of both workouts; strength training and cardio. According to recent studies, kettlebells is ranked at *20 calories a minute* in terms of calorie-burns. It takes into account both the aerobic and the anaerobic calorie expenditure. You have to realize that very few cardio exercises contribute to muscle building, but kettlebells are an exception. With this, you can burn between *500-600 calories in just half an hour, incredible!*

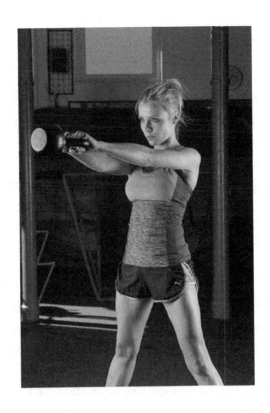

For someone who is able to do about 50 reps of any exercise, there is a high probability that you are not using the kettlebells exercise to your advantage. You are not supposed to go light on this exercise if this is you. Either way, do not go too heavy as well. Some of the very best ways in which you can maximize losing calories is doing this for about 45 minutes and then resting for 20 minutes. Keep repeating this cycle as many times as you can. Set your time at 30 minutes intervals and see how far you can go and how much calories you can get off.

Jumping Rope

There are so many reasons why jumping rope is not a kid's thing but is a mainstay even among boxer trainers. Not only is very cheap, but also easy to do, increases the speed of the foot while burning tons of calories. Imagine your favorite boxer, fighter or wrestler-the truth is they all jump roles. This exercise does not only improve your footwork, strength of the shoulder and coordination, but also is a simulation of sprinting. It allows you to lose as much as *500 calories in just half an hour*.

The best way to make the most of this exercise is by doing intervals of fast and slow jumps as far as you can go. If you cannot do that so well, then you can jump as fast as you can for a minute, then rest 30 seconds before you can resume. Keep repeating these cycles until you are done. If you travel frequently, throw a skipping rope in your travel bag for a great workout experience at the comfort of your hotel room. You will thank me for it later :)

Stair climber

This is one of the most popular ways in which you can burn tons of fats and calories at a moderate pace. The higher leg lift involved in this exercise ensures that when climbing the stairs, you use more muscles as compared to those involved during walking. The truth is, strengthening your legs is important and you achieve this in a functional way using this exercise. However, it is important to take note that this exercise comes with a significant drawback as the stair climbers can concentrate so much weight and pressure on the joints, hence making it quite difficult for people with bad knees to manage.

The best way to get the most of this workout is by incorporating about 90% or more effort on the stair climber for half a minute with about a minute recovery. When you do about 20-15 rounds of this exercise, you are sure to have a well spiced up workout and burn more calories above the normal range.

Elliptical

This is a machine that was designed to minimize the impact that hits your hips and knees while still helping you have a great workout. Considering the fact that the impact is low, the calorie burning effect is not that high. This means that unlike other machines like treadmills, the impact that you get from this machine is not that great. However, if you are just starting out, it can be great to help bring your body to speed before you can adopt a more vigorous option like a treadmill.

You can use this machine to lose weight gradually without necessarily wearing out your joints. With an Elliptical, an average man of about *180 lbs.* may lose between *500-600 calories/hour* if they are going at moderate pace. To get more out of this, you can decide to switch the intensity, resistance and speed settings.

The best way you can use the Elliptical to burn fat is by adding a high incline on it so that you can activate more leg muscles and most specifically, the glutes. You can also have a cross-country feel with it if you lower the incline and increase resistance to really work your quads. One thing though, when using this machine, please do not hold on too tightly to the handles or rails as with step mill since this can significantly reduce your efforts and might end up with pain on your shoulders and wrist.

Running

Here I'm talking about running at a steady moderate pace. This is one of the sure ways in which you can burn as much calories as you can. However, it is not the most economical way to build up or even maintain your muscles. By running, an average person of about *180 lbs.* can burn up to *950 calories/hour* while running at a pace of *8.5 min/mile.*

An important point to note is that running at this pace may break down your muscles and subject your body to compounding. Therefore, if you are looking to include this long run into your routine every often, it is better to opt for the trails or softer surfaces rather than cement.

If you are running using a treadmill, then it is recommended that you set that incline to 2-3% so that you can adequately simulate a run outside. This will ensure that you burn more calories while going easy on your knees. If you find running to be a little easy, then you can try different routes in the neighborhood or try running with a group of friends, family or joining a running club. You will be amazed how far you go and how long you can actually go without noticing. It simply makes the miles go easier!

Chapter 4

Weight Training

The greatest advantage that you get when working out with weights is the fact that is addition to shedding off a couple of pounds, you build your muscles. It is these muscles that burn calories. This is one of the best healthy feedback loops that you can get. According to experts, working all your major muscle groups at least three times every week goes a long way in helping you keep that weight off.

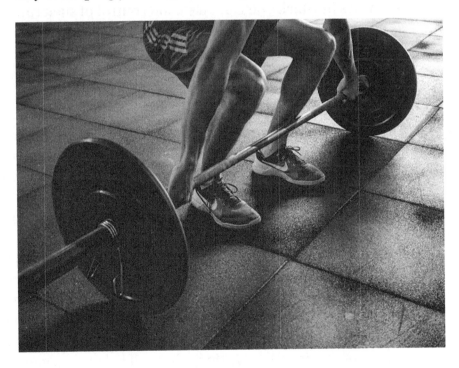

So, what are the benefits of Weight Training?

There are so many benefits that you can reap from weight training apart from losing weight. Anything that helps you get the weight off and still adds you more advantage is worth your while, right?

Well, not only does weight training increase your physical work capacity, but also boosts your capability to activities of daily living, also referred to as ADL's. In other words, with weight training, you can work harder for longer durations as long as you have the right weight training activities.

Secondly, weight training plays a critical role in helping you improve your bone density. In other words, it is one of the best ways in which you can take good control of such things as bone loss which happens a lot as one progresses with age. It simply adds a lot of strength on the bones and you can achieve this by integrating strength training in your workout plans.

Thirdly, weight training helps promote a fat free body mass. Did you know that your lean body mass that we all work so hard for often decreases with increase in age? Well, now you do. If you add weight training into your weight loss management plan, then you will be able to burn all that fat.

Fourthly, weight training contributes a lot to the strength of your muscles, connective tissues as well as tendons. This plays a significant role in improving the motor performance and hence reducing the risk for injury. With all these benefits, it is safe to say that weight training generally improves your quality of life. It is the one thing that will help you regain your body confidence. It will not only make you strong, but also offer you a good alternative to managing your weight.

Exercises

Here are some of the exercises that you can engage in at least every week in half-hour sessions. For each of these exercises, begin with a set of about 8-10 repetitions during the first two weeks. When you are choosing what weight to use, you have to bear in mind that the last 3-4 repetitions have to be very difficult. In the coming weeks after that, you can increase the reps to about 15 and gradually work your way up to make the most of these exercises and shed off as much weight as possible within the shortest time possible.

When performing these repetitions, you will realize that they become a little easier overtime. This means that you have to keep making it difficult each time so that they are effective in helping you lose as many calories as you can. You can achieve this by lifting heavier weights. Ensure that during the process, you are taking deep breaths. This is by exhaling during the exertion/lifting stage and inhaling as you bring the weight down.

Dumbbell chest fly

This exercise often targets the chest. Begin by lying on your back ensuring that you have support on your shoulders head and your upper back. Then hold the dumbbell; in each hand. You start with dumbbells of between 2-5 pounds in weight.

Begin to push your arms straight up or until your elbows are almost fully extended and your palms are facing each other. It is very important that you ensure that your weight is directly above your shoulders. Then inhale and slowly lower your arms out to the side ensuring that your elbows are bent just slightly.

Keep lowering your arms until your elbows are just slightly below your shoulders. Keep it there and exhale. Then slowly close your arms back to your starting position.

Dumbbell overheads triceps extensions

This exercise specifically targets the triceps as the name suggests. With this exercise, begin by standing on your feet so that your shoulder-width is apart. Hold a dumbbell on each one of your hands ensuring that each one of your arms is extended overhead. Again, here you can start with 2-5 pounds dumbbells and begin to work your way up.

Without moving your elbows, lower the right dumbbell very slowly so that it is positioned behind your neck. Pause at that position and then begin to lift it to your starting position. Repeat the same with the left hand.

Dumbbell shoulder press

This exercise specifically targets the shoulders. Begin by first sitting on a chair with your back fully supported and that your feet are flat on the floor. Hold your dumbbells on each of your hands and just like I have mentioned earlier, if you are starting out, you should begin with 2-5 pounds dumbbells and work your way up gradually.

Slowly bend your arms so that the weight rests lightly on your shoulders while ensuring that your palms are facing forward. Then begin to push the weights up slowly until your arms are straight. Pause for a second in that position and then slowly return to your starting position.

Single leg squat

This is a very great exercises that targets most parts of your body including the buttocks, calves and the quadriceps. To start this exercise, begin by standing on your feet ensuring that the shoulder-width is apart and your arms are out to the sides and raised to the height of your shoulders.

Slowly lift your legs out in front of you and then slowly squat down. At this point, it is important that I mention that, if you feel like you are losing your balance, you should stop for a minute before giving it another try. However, if you are close to a wall and you need balancing, you could achieve this by placing one hand on the wall.

Once you have your balance, then begin to contract your legs and buttock muscles so that you can push yourself back to your starting position. Complete all your reps and then switch your legs and start over again.

Chin up

Did you know that chins are one of the most basic ways in which you can effectively burn those calories and gain a muscle mass? This is because, when doing this exercise, you are forced to use as many muscle groups and the curl the weight of your body.

To perform this exercise, begin by grasping the chin up bar while ensuring that your shoulder-width achieve a supinated grip in such a way that your palms are upward facing. Allow your body to hang on the bar with your arms fully stretched straight. Slowly, begin to pull yourself up in such a way that your chin is much higher than the bar. With controlled movements, start lowering your body to its starting position.

To make the most of this exercise, it is important that you ensure your feet are in line with your torso throughout the entire exercise. Secondly, ensure that your arms are fully extended at the very bottom of the exercise prior to transitioning to the next repetition. Also, hold the dumbbells between your feet to achieve an additional resistance.

Bent over row

This is also referred to as Barbell rows. This is one of the best back exercises that you can get in order to burn body fats and build muscle mass. Just like many other row variations, this exercise targets specifically the lats as well as the upper back muscle, the shoulders and the biceps. In order to get the most of the exercise, you have to ensure that you keep your back straight and your feet firmly rooted on the floor throughout the duration of the exercise. Ensure that you focus on pulling your shoulder blades together while rowing the weight.

To get started, place your feet a shoulder apart at the front of the loaded barbell. Then bend over the bar just so that you are parallel with the floor. Grasp the bar with a wider grip than the shoulder width apart. Slowly begin to lift the bar up until it is above the ground while keeping your back as straight as you can and your knees are bent.

Now, with a clean controlled motion, begin to raise the bar towards your chest by simply contracting your arms and slowly pulling the shoulder blades towards each other until they meet. Keep doing this until the bar is in touch with your lower chest. Pause for a second before you can return the bar to its original starting position. You can do this by extending your arms slowly and then lowering the weight.

Some of the tips to help you make the most of this exercise is concentration on maintaining a good posture throughout the exercise. Also, keep your back as straight as you can throughout the exercise period while ensuring that your feet are firmly planted on the ground. Pay a closer attention on squeezing your shoulder blades together as a row. Perform each row slowly and in a controlled manner just by using your arms and back.

Pull ups

These are one of the most common and beneficial weight loss exercises. Unfortunately, most people fail at it because they are a great test of strength. However, if you try and are not able to complete a set of pull ups, build your strength with chin ups and other alternatives that work best for you especially if you are just getting started.

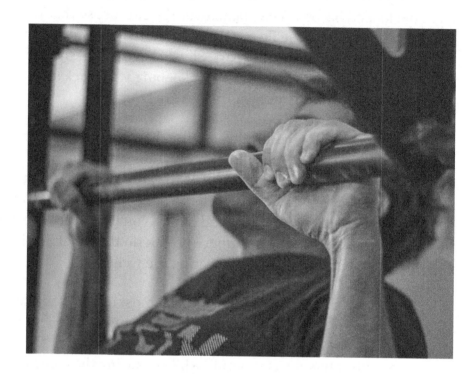

To perform this exercise, the first thing that you have to do is to grab the bar with an overhand grip that is much wider than the shoulder width apart. Then allow your torso to hang straight down. This will be your starting position.

Then begin by pulling your torso up by simply allowing your arms to contract in such a way that your shoulders as well as the upper arms are drawn down and back. Continue to pull upwards until the bar comes in contact with your upper chest.

Then take a pause for about a second or two before inhaling and returning to your starting position, by simply extending your arms and lowering your torso. Keep repeating this for the required number of times that you have defined to make a set.

Some of the most important tips that will help you make the most of this exercise is concentrating very closely on squeezing the back muscles at the top of the lift. Ensure that while at it, you keep the back as straight as you can throughout the entire duration of the exercise. Perform each repetition in each set in a very slow and controlled manner with the help of your arms and your back. Just remember to keep your back straight.

Power clean

This is one of the easiest ones of the weight training exercises. In order to achieve your weight loss goals and attain health and fitness, it is important that you add this exercise into your weight loss plan/routine as it concentrates on engaging your upper body and the lower body as well. This exercise targets the hamstrings, quadriceps, traps, lower back, forearms, glutes, calves as well as the upper back.

To perform this exercise, the first thing that you have to do is to place the loaded barbell on the ground in front of you. Then stand with your feet rooted on the ground so that they are shoulder width apart over the bar. Ensure that while you establish your starting position, your toes are pointing forward below the bar.

Then squat down and hold the bar by simply bending your knees in such a way that your hamstrings and your quadriceps are parallel to the floor. Your arms and back should be straight and your chest pointing upwards. Another thing is for you to ensure that you have an overhand grip that is shoulder width apart or wider than this just slightly. Now, this is your starting position.

Now, it is time to begin the exercise by simply deadlifting the bar upwards. You can do this by simply pressing from your heels and then extending your hips and knees. Ensure that while doing this, your back is straight and it maintains the same angle while you lift the weight. As the bar reaches the level of your knees, extend your hips, ankles and knees explosively in a jumping motion so that the bar moves upwards a fast pace.

As the bar raises, you can try to shrug your shoulders just a little while pulling the bar upwards to allow your elbows to flex out to the sides. Use the weight's momentum in order to pull your boarder more aggressively under the bar while rotating the elbows under the bar. Then slowly allow the weight to land on your shoulders while ensuring that you move into the front squat position.

Once at the bottom of the front squat, ensure that your hamstrings as well as the quadriceps are parallel to the floor and then immediately stand up and press upwards while extending your knees and hips.

To make the most of this exercise, you have to take note of very important tips. Remember that this is a more advanced exercise that should only be performed with limited amount of weight. This is especially true at the beginning until you are well adjusted to every stage of the exercise. You have to also bear in mind that this is not an exercise that is recommended for people with lower back problems. In as much as you would like to lose that extra pound so fast, your safety has to come first. When you get to the jumping movement, this is your main generator for energy and not your shoulders and arms pulling the bar upwards.

Chest dips

This is a body weight exercise that is plays a very important role in burning fats around the chest areas. It is a slight variation of the Triceps dips. You may be thinking 'how are these exercises different?' Well, during lifting, you lean forward to achieve an angle of about 30°. Then you flare out your elbows while lowering your body. With this exercise, you will also use the bars angled outwards and they have to be slightly wider than the bars used in Tricep dips.

To perform this exercise, you have to be at the gym dip station. You then hold your body in such a way that they are at arm's length above the bars. It is important that you look for bars that are angled outwards and are slightly wider than what people typically use for Triceps dips. Under usual circumstances, you will find that the station comprises a set of parallel bars for triceps dips and another separate set of bars for the chest dip.

Then begin to lean forward to about an angle of 30° and then breath in while slowly lowering your torso by bending at the elbows so that they can flare out just a little. Remember to lower your body just until your triceps are parallel to the bars. Or until you feel your chest stretch a little.

Then breath out while pushing your body back up slowly to your starting position. Ensure that you are doing this while concentrating on your chest. Then squeeze your chest at the top of the movement for just a second or two. Then repeat this movement for the set number of repetitions making up a set.

In order to make the most of the chest dips, ensure that, if you are not strong enough to complete this exercise, you should build up your strength by simply doing the negatives especially using the dip machine or even a weight assisted dip machine. You could also use a spotter to help hold your feet in position during the exercise. Ensure that you make the exercise quite challenging by attaching weight plate to a weighted belt or by just holding a dumbbell between your feel.

Concentrate so much on utilizing your chest to complete the weight lifting while ensuring that you squeeze the pecs at the very top of the movement.

Leg press exercise

This is an exercise that does not make use of free weights. It often targets all the major muscles on the legs. It also achieves this by simply using a weight machine while allowing you to pile on the weight.

To perform the exercise, begin by slightly adjusting the seat machine so that your feet fits comfortably and achieves a crosspiece position with the knees bent slightly. Then start pressing your feet forward at the shoulder width stance. Then slowly release the safety locks.

Next, start lowering the weight towards your body while ensuring that you keep your abs drawn in and the knees moving in one direction as the feet in such a way that they are all at a right-angle orientation. Then push the weight forward slowly by extending your legs. Press upwards so that you ensure that the weights are equally distributed between your forefoot and the heel. Then finally lower the weight slowly to its starting position. Repeat this for the entire number of reps there is in a set. Just make sure that you do not lock your knees or bounce the weight fast during the exercise.

Food for thought- Safe and effective weight training

Did you know that so many people do the same routine in the exact order for decades? Well, the truth is, it can be quite comforting to master your weight loss program, but the main problem kicks in when your muscles adapt and get bored, and you will get bored as well.

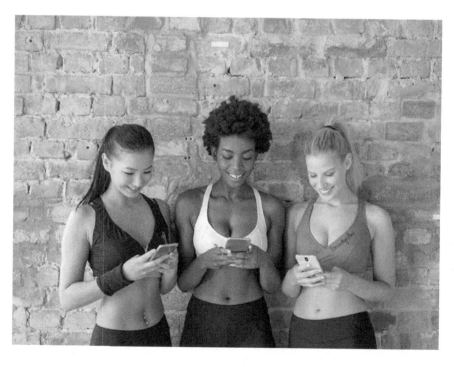

Therefore, if you are going to lose weight, you have to keep tweaking your weight training routine every often. You can change such things as the number of reps, angles, rest periods, sequence of events as well as the type of equipment that you use. Also, it is important that you keep the following tips in mind at all times to ensure that you stay safe and make the most out of each workout.

Never skip a warm-up session !

For so many people, they want to lose weight straight away and so they think that they can just go straight from the locker room into doing the bench press. The truth is, even though your main aim is to lose weight immediately, your body may get overwhelmed at everything. <u>You need to bring your body to a state that is ready for more vigorous exercise</u>. The best way in which you can achieve this is by warming up before starting any session.

To warm up your muscles, you can start with aerobic exercises which are absolutely great for your cardio. Also, it is important that you go easy on the very first set of each strength training exercise just to ensure that the body has the right momentum to keep up.

Do not allow the momentum to do the work

One of the things that you have to bear in mind is that if you lift weights so fats you are simply allowing your body to develop momentum. This means that you are allowing the body the make exercising quite easy on the muscles. One thing is that so many people are kind of laxed especially when it can come to the return phase of a lift. In other words, they will host the dumbbells up slowly and then let them come down so fast!

To ensure that you guard against this, take at least two seconds to lift, and then pause for a second or two at the top before you take another two seconds to bring the weight down to its starting position.

Do not hold your breathe

When you are lifting the weight up, it is very important that you remember to take a deep breathe. This is because, you need lots of oxygen when lifting. When you hold your breath or take in shallow breathes, you may end up elevating your blood pressure and zapping your energy. Therefore, just take the time to breathe through your mouth rather than using your nose that you take in as much oxygen as possible.

For many kinds of exercises, ensure that you exhale when lifting the weights up and then inhale when lowering it down. On the other hand, for those that expand the chest cavity, it is natural to inhale as you lift the weight up and exhale when releasing it to the starting position.

Mix up

In order for you to keep making gains, you have to ensure that change your routine every often as mentioned earlier. For example, you can increase the amount of weight you are lifting or increase the number of repeats by 10% each time or lower your rest time between sets.

All these adjustments play a very important in ensuring that you burn as much calories as you can. You may be thinking 'but how many repetitions are enough?' Well, the truth is, you should be lifting enough weight so that the last two-three repetitions are quite challenging and reduce the rest time between each set. For many people, having about 12-15 repetitions can be enough but you have to work to increase them every often so that the exercises are challenging enough and you burn more calories per set.

With good weight training routine, you may end up seeing results in just a few weeks. Ensure that you keep up your effort so that you have more defined muscles, achieve a better balance and lose enough weight to improve your overall health and looks!

Chapter 5

Yoga

Did you know that yoga is one of the most intense exercises that can help you to lose that weight and keep it off? Well, now you know! Based on a recent study conducted by Fred Hutchinson Cancer Research Center, people who practice yoga and mindfulness regularly often live it as a lifestyle. They pay a close attention to what they eat and hence, are less likely to be obese. So, what is going to be like for you in 2019?

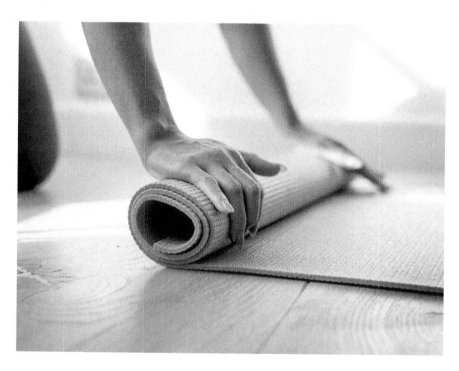

Well, while Yoga is considered traditionally as an aerobic exercise, there are some kinds of yoga that are more physical.

The types of yoga that are intense play a central role in ensuring that you burn more calories. Apart from trimming off that weight, yoga also plays a critical role in helping you develop muscle tone as well as boost metabolism.

Despite the fact that restorative yoga is not a physical kind of yoga, it is essential in weight loss. According to research, there is evidence showing that restorative yoga is very effective in helping women lose weight especially around the abdomen. It is these findings that are very promising for people like you who want to lose weight fast. In another study conducted in 2013, there is evidence that shows yoga as a promising way to alter one's behavior, help them lose weight as well as maintain it by burning calories. This also heightens one's mindfulness and helps reduce stress levels. Because of these factors, you will be able to reduce the amount of food that you eat as well as become self-aware of effects associated with overeating.

Let's look at some Yoga exercises that you can incorporate into your weight loss routine/plan.

Prasarita Padottanasana

This is also referred to as wide-legged forward bend. To practice this, the first thing that you have to do is ensure that your hands are touching the floor in front of you. While in this pose, ensure that you add in an extra shoulder stretch.

Then begin to spread your feet to about 4 feet apart. Bend forward slowly at the hips and NOT the waist. Ensure that while doing this, your back is as straight as possible without hunching forward. If you are bending properly, you should feel a strong stretch in your hamstrings. You can practice this in front of the mirror until you can be able to get it right.

Then hold it in that position for about 6 breaths. If you are comfortable enough, you could clasp your hands behind your back. Then try as much as you can to bring them forward towards the ceiling so that your arms and shoulders help you get that extra stretch.

Anjaneyasana

This is also referred to as a lunge. This exercise is one of the best poses that you can use to stretch your hips. So many people often tend to have very tight hips because of sitting for prolonged hours in front of a computer. Not only will this exerciser help increase flexibility for the splits but also help you achieve stretched lips if that is one of your main goals as well.

You have to bear in mind that your hands can be wherever you need them to be while doing asana. The location of your arms often is a determining factor of what muscles you are trying to stretch. If you raise your arms up and slightly tilt them backwards, you will be able to bring the stretch into the back and the hips. You could also bring your arms down to the sides and slightly behind in order for you to stretch your lower back.

The third option is to allow your arms rest on your knees in front of you, despite the fact that you may not be able to achieve much of a stretch on the hips. Whatever option you chose to go with, it is important for you to ensure that your front knees are a at a right angle as much as you possibly can.

Then hold that position for about a minute before you repeat it on the other side.

Ardha Navasana

This is also referred to as half boat pose. This is a great yoga asana that plays a large role in weight loss. This is because it directly works on your tummy! With this exercise, you will feel as though your abs muscles are working hard while trying to hold this pose.

Then put your arms down onto the ground in order to achieve a balance. Then begin to raise your legs first. Once you feel that you have adequate stability, slowly raise your arms so that they are parallel with the ground.

However, if you feel that this is not challenging enough, try increasing the space between your knees as well as the chest. This you can achieve by simply leaning back slightly and then moving your knees just further from you just a little. When doing this, you should be able to feel your abs burning, indicating that you are doing it right.

Hold that position for a minute. If you feel very comfortable in this pose, try as much as you can to straighten your legs so that you get an extra challenge. Now, this is a full boat pose and I bet you can already learn that is quite hard to balance in.

Vasisthasana

This is also referred to as a side plank. This explains the reason why this form of "plank" made it to the top list of yoga asana as it plays a central role in helping people lose weight. This plank among other variations are very important in working your abs.

When you are in a regular plank position with your palms facing down on a yoga mat and the shoulder width apart with toes together on the mat, begin to tilt your feet in such a manner that the outer right side of your right foot is in contact with the mat. This also ensures that your left foot is on top of the right foot.

Then start shifting your weight onto your right hand as you remove your left hand from the mat. Then lift your left arm slowly with your head straight up towards the ceiling. Ensure that your hips and shoulders are stacked in this pose. In other words, they should be in direct line with one another and not leaning towards the back. Keep this position for about a minute and then repeat it on the other side.

Vriksasana

This is also referred to as tree pose. Well, so many people think that this pose is quite easy, but trust me, It's harder to balance in this pose than you may think.

To exercise it, begin by bringing your foot to rest on the inside of your left thigh. Ensure that while at it, your back is kept straight as you possibly can. You will realize that your body will tend to bend forward when you are trying to balance, but even so, try as much as you can to bring your shoulder back up every time.

Now try to keep your hands pressed together at your heart. This is very important in ensuring that you can balance. Once you have a balance, try lifting your hands above your head so that your hands are directly pointed towards the ceiling. Hold that position for a minute before changing and repeating with the other side as well.

Parivrtta anjaneyasana

This is also referred to as revolved lunge pose. With this exercise, you can keep your right hands on the floor next to the left foot so that you get your support when getting into the pose. Try as much as you can to keep your front knee at a right angle bend so that your overstretched legs are straight.

Then bring your right elbow forward so that it rests on your left knee. Then bring both your hands together. Press the hands into each other so that you increase the stretch both in the shoulders and your back. Start tightening your core while maintaining this pose so that you work your abs so more. Hold it at that position for about 6 breaths or for a minute before you can repeat the same for the other side.

Utkatasana

This is also referred to as chair pose. In other words, it is the yoga version of a squat hold. It deserves a spot on the yoga asana list for weight loss. With this exercise, you will be able to work your quadriceps as much as you can. Keep your feet together and your arms as straight as you can so that they are above you when you try lowering your body to a squatting position.

While doing this, ensure that you can see your feet in front of your knees. However, if you are not able to, try to adjust your feet into position because they may be bent too far forward. Try as much as you can to tuck your hips in a little to avoid arching your back too much.

Then try to get your thighs in position so that they are parallel to the ground without necessarily compromising your position and form. Hold that position for a minute.

Virabhadrasana I

This exercise is often performed as a flow. In other words, you perform the exercise from one pose to another pose in a fluid manner. The warrior routine is a very critical component of the yoga asana for weight loss and should not be overlooked at all.

The warrior I is quite similar to high lunge. However, with this exercise, the back foot is pointed out at an angle instead of being tucked under the foot. When doing this exercise, you have to ensure that you keep your front knee at a right angle. However, if you are a beginner, your stance may be slightly higher than 90°.

Once you achieve this posture, try to maintain that pose for a minute before you can change to Warrior II. Also, ensure that you repeat this as a vinyasa using the other side of your body once you are done with the first side.

Virabhadrasana II

This is also referred to as Warrior II. From the Warrior I pose that we just discussed above, you are required to extend your arms to the sides so that you can move your chest as well as the hips to face a similar direction as your back foot.

Once again, with this exercise, it is important that you keep the front knees at a right angle as much as you possibly can. Ensure that your arms are parallel to the ground. Then hold that pose for a minute before you can change it to Warrior III. Once you are done, you can repeat all three poses on the other side of the body.

Virabhadrasana III

This is also referred to as Warrior III. This is the most difficult one of all the three vinyasa. Well, so many people think that it is quite easy at first, but once they start exercising it, they realize how hard it is to hold this pose with the right form for more than a minute.

Once you are done with Warrior II, try to twist your chest so that it faces towards the forward direction. Then start bringing your arms out in such a way that they are straight and point in front of you to achieve a balanced pose.

If you are a yoga beginner, you might have to bring your back leg so close to the front so that you have a balance before you can start lifting it. Then start bringing your pals together so that they are at your chest as you start lifting up your leg into the air. This is because it plays a significant role in helping achieve a tremendous balance.

Once you are in the right position, raise your arms slowly so that they are both out in front of you. Ensure that while you are doing this, your back toes are pointed to achieve the right pose. The truth is, if you are a beginner, it might take time flexibility and strength before you can actually get it right. Therefore, ensure that you keep practicing in front of a mirror until you have it right. Once you do, hold that pose for a minute and then repeat the whole vinyasa from I through II to III using the other side of your body.

Chapter 6

The 4-Week Full-Body Workout And 12-Week Diet Plan

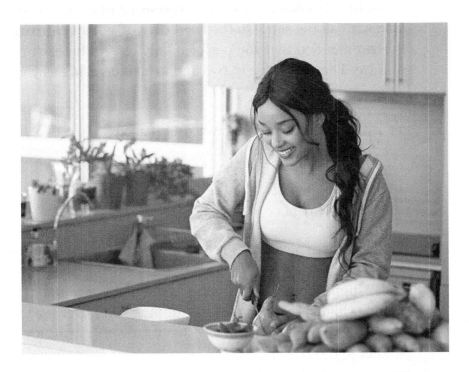

When trying to lose weight over the shortest time possible, you have to blend a diet and workout plan that works best to support your goals. This means that you have to perform the workout at least three days every week for at least a month. You also have to ensure that you rest at least a day in between the workout sessions.

In the case of weight exercises, it is important that you choose weights that allow you to complete a number of reps more than the number that is prescribed. For example, if the exercise calls for about 11 reps, you could choose to do 15 reps instead. Also, it is important that you perform these reps in pairs. In this case, I have marked them as A and B where necessary so that you can alternate between each set and taking at least a minute to rest between the sets.

In other words, if you start with A, you complete it before you can switch to B. however, before you proceed to B, you have to rest in between. You will keep repeating this until you are done with all the sets. On the **first day of your training**, it is recommended that you perform only one set for each exercise. Then progress to two and keep increasing as your body also adjusts to these changes.

Let's start with the 4-Week workout plan.

1 Front Squat

This comprises of 3 sets, 8 reps and a rest of about a minute in between. Now, I would like you to get started with barbell on the support of a power rack. Ensure that it is about a shoulder high. Then proceed to grabbing a bar overhead and raise your elbows in such a way that your upper arms are parallel to the ground.

Proceed by lifting the bar off the rack and then allow it to roll towards your fingers. This is the position you should allow it to rest throughout the duration of the whole exercise. Remember that, if you keep your elbows in position, you will not have to struggle with having a balance. Squat as low as you possibly can and then begin to drive with your legs so that you can return to your original position. Now, this is one rep. Repeat this for the number of reps you desire.

2A: Three-point Dumbbell row

This one comprises of 3 sets, 15 reps per arm and a rest duration of a minute. Start by grabbing the dumbbell using your left hand. Then rest your right hand on a flat bench so that you have a support that gives you balance. While doing this, ensure that your back is kept as straight as possible and your shoulders are in line with the floor. Begin to row the weight up to your chest.

Now, lower your dumbbell so that you can get back to your starting position. That is one rep. repeat this for the desired number of reps alternating between your right hand and the left hand every time.

2B: Push ups

This exercise comprises of 3 sets with 18 reps and a rest duration of about a minute. Start by placing your hands on the ground or a floor mat so that you are a about shoulder width apart and well stretched. Then extend your legs straight on your back so that your body forms a straight line from your head to your heels. Then lower your body in such a way that your torso is an inch off the ground/floor mat. Push yourself back up slowly. This makes one rep. Repeat this for the number of reps you desire.

3A: Single-leg bridge

This comprises of 3 sets and 15 reps separated by a rest duration of about one minute. Start by lying on a floor mat with your back. Now, bend one of your knees in such a manner that that your foot is flat on the floor mat. Ensure that you keep the opposite leg as straight on the floor as possible. Then start pushing your foot into the floor and then raise your hips until both your thighs are parallel to each other. Slowly reverse this motion so that you get back to your original starting position. Now, that is one rep. Complete the other remaining reps by switching your legs every time.

3B: Dumbbell Pullover

This exercise is comprised of 3 sets with 15 reps and a rest duration of about 60 seconds. To perform this, start by holding one dumbbell with both your hands and then lie down with your back resting on the bench. Begin to slowly press the dumbbell straight over your face. Lower your arms so that they are behind your head. Do this as far as you can go and then pull back the dumbbell to its original position. That makes one rep. Complete the other number of reps.

4: Plank

This comprises of 3 sets and the reps lasts for a minute each with 60 seconds rest periods between reps. To get started, get yourself into a push-up position and then begin to bend your elbows so that they are in a right angle. Then rest your weight on your forearms while keeping the rest of your body in a straight line. Hold at that position for a minute. That is one set. Now, repeat this for the desired number of sets.

The 12 Week Diet Plan

For a weight loss meal plan, it is important that you have at least three different types of eating days that include;

High carb days comprising a day/week

Moderate carb days comprising about 3 days a week

Low carb days comprising about 3 days a week

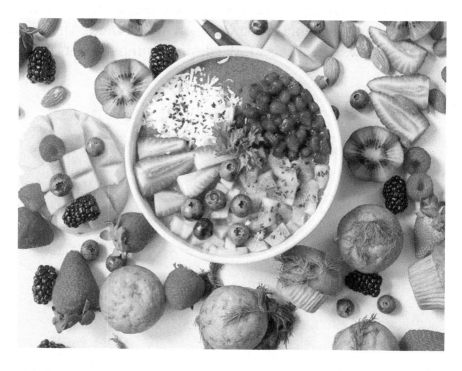

You have to ensure that you structure the days in the best way possible so that they suit your preference. This means that, for high carb days, just keep them for special occasions. For instance, you may be attending a family dinner, eating out with friends or even indulging a little with your partner.

You have to note that the calorie intake is adjustable based on metabolism. For instance

Men within the age of 40 and above should reduce their calorie intake by 300

Men between 20-25 years of age should increase their calorie intake by 300

Women within the age of 40 and above should reduce their calorie intake by 200

Women between the age of 20-25 above should increase their calorie intake by 200

Weeks	Low Carb Days	Moderate Carbs Days	High Carb Day
Week 1	3 low carb days with 2300 calories	3 moderate carbs days with 2400 calories	1 high carb day of 2700 calories
Week 2	3 low carb days with 2200 calories	3 moderate carbs days with 2400	1 high carb day of 2700 calories
Week 3	3 low carb days with 2100 calories	3 moderate carbs days with 2400	1 high carb day of 2700 calories
Week 4	3 low carb days with 2000 calories	3 moderate carbs days with 2400 calories	high carb day of 2700 calories
Week 5	3 low carb days with 2300 calories	3 moderate carbs days with 2300	1 high carb day of 2700 calories
Week 6	3 low carb days with 2200 calories	3 moderate carbs days with 2300	1 high carb day of 2700 calories
Week 7	3 low carb days with 2100 calories	3 moderate carbs days with 2300	1 high carb day of 2700 calories
Week 8	3 low carb days with 2000 calories	3 moderate carbs days with 2300	1 high carb day of 2700 calories
Week 9	3 low carb days with 2300 calories	3 moderate carbs days with 2200	1 high carb day of 2700 calories
Week 10	3 low carb days with 2200 calories	3 moderate carbs days with 2200	1 high carb day of 2700 calories
Week 11	3 low carb days with 2100 calories	3 moderate carbs days with 2200	1 high carb day of 2700 calories
Week 12	3 low carb days with 2000 calories	3 moderate carbs days with 2200	1 high carb day of 2700 calories

12 Week Eating Plan

If you are going to lose weight, you have to ensure that your minimum protein intake per day is at 150-180 grams. However, if you are a bigger guy and have a fair muscle mass, then you should at least consume 180-200 grams. This is because, if you eat lots of proteins then you have to drop your fat intake to make up for the calories. Your fat intake should be between 20-30% of daily calories. You have your calorie intake in check, then fill in with healthy carbs.

The 12 Week Cardio Plan

The truth is, irrespective of what cardio you use for the 12 weeks, what is important is for you to select exercises that gets you heart beating. It can be elliptical, treadmill or swimming. The first thing that you will realize with this cardio plan is that it starts at a slow rate and that is perfectly fine. This is because, at this point, you are out of shape and you need the body to start acclimatizing to these changes in workouts so that you gain proper momentum for vigorous exercises.

This workout plan is designed so that you get back in shape within 12 weeks. The thing with losing weight is that patience is key. Trust the plan and stick to it. Once the 12 weeks are gone, you will be surprised at how much weight you have lost.

In this book, we have seen so many exercises that you can perform in order to shed off that weight. Well, this plan here is just a warm up plan and you can incorporate the other exercises by spreading them through the weeks.

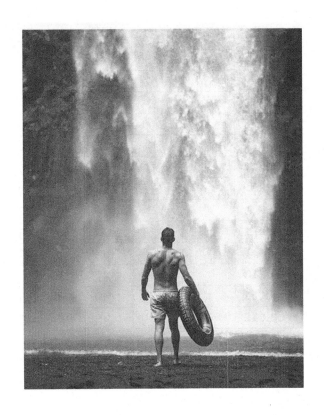

Week	Cardio Session	Reps	Duration
Week 1	3	5	5
Week 2	3	8	8
Week 3	3	10	10
Week 4	3	12	12
Week 5	3	15	15
Week 6	3	20	20
Week 7	4	20	22
Week 8	4	22	25
Week 9	4	25	27
Week 10	4	27	30
Week 11	4	30	35
Week 12	4	35	45

Chapter 7

Conclusion

We have discussed the various ways in which you can lose weight fast. Well whether your main goal is to shed off 10 pounds or 100 pounds, it is important to note that the weight loss journey is a great undertaking that is accompanied by lots of challenges. However, the good thing is that you are strong enough to look at the brighter side of things- **regaining control of your body!**

Contrary to so many myths about diets that people belief in, the truth is, for you to lose weight. You do not have to starve yourself. If you are going to work every morning, rather than getting caught in a trap of having to eat unhealthy snacks, it is better if you carried your own snack. This way, you will not have to hit the vending machine for those potato chips.

The other thing is, in most cases, people get to bad eating habits because they attend events with friends and they can't help but indulge or should I say-Overindulge? Well, you have to think active if you are going to burn those calories. You can also take a dance class, take a walk or surround yourself with people that will appreciate what you are trying to achieve and support you every step of the way.

Portion control can be a great issue when it comes to weight loss. To overcome the temptation of eating so much calories than required, it is better if you stock up your foods in containers so that you get everything in the correct portion.

For every step that you make, it is important that you reward yourself with something other than food! There are so many things you can do like getting that new workout outfit you have been admiring. The truth is, unlike food rewards, this will help you have a different perspective of fitness as a fun activity rather than a punishment.

The other thing is that not all people are going to support you through your slimming journey. So many people will be jealous of your decision to lose weight and will try as much as they can to ridicule you. Rather than giving up and letting them take control of what decisions you make, *spend time with people who will cheer you on no matter what.* Always keep your eye on the prize-a healthy body weight and shape!

So many people get into weight lose plan and at first things are slow and when they begin to peak up, they realize that they are adding weight rather than shedding it. Well, this can be discouraging, but the truth is, it is absolutely normal! You have to keep pushing past it by increasing the intensity of your workouts and watching your calorie-intake very closely. Ensure that you make vegetables your friend. This is because they are very high in nutrients and low in calories.

Finally, bear in mind that not having a plan in itself is planning to for failure. Therefore, plan everything including your workouts, diets and grocery lists in advance so that you do not fail. Also, remember that losing weight lowers the risk for a number of serious diseases, helps you sleep better, boosts your relationship and boosts your confidence too. Therefore, losing weight with all these in mind is worth everything. *Just don't give up on the dream !*

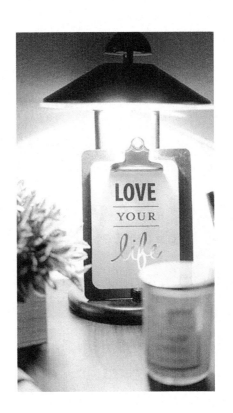

About Author

Gabrielle Hollis

Gabrielle Hollis is a Fitness Expert,

decluttering specialist, blogger and lifestyle designer.

She lives in North Carolina with her husband and three kids.

She has worked with thousands of people throughout her career.

Gabrielle is an author of books which help solve problems with diet,

workouts, losing weight, messy home, life and relationships.

Made in the USA
Middletown, DE
21 January 2022